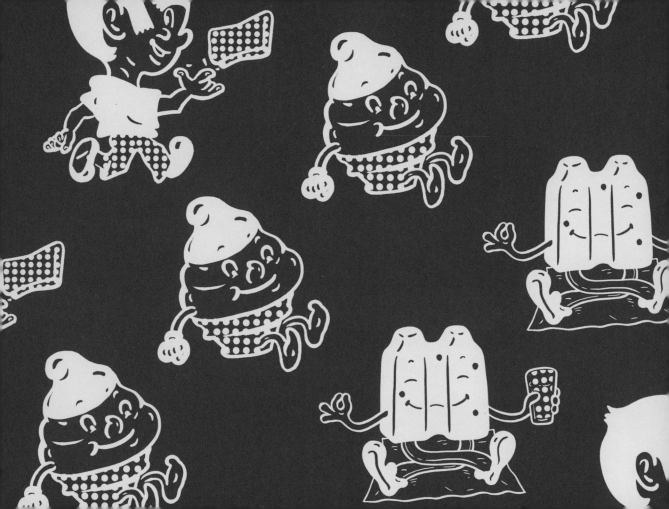

VINNIE'S CRAMP KICKING REMEDIES

AND OTHER CLEVER CURES FOR PMS, BLOATING, AND MORE!

BY VINNIE

CHRONICLE BOOKS
SAN FRANCISCO

Library of Congress Cataloging-in-Publication Data available.
ISBN: 0-8118-4249-5

Manufactured in China.

Design by Alethea Morrison.

Distributed in Canada by Raincoast Books
9050 Shaughnessy Street
Vancouver, British Columbia V6P 6E5

Chronicle Books LLC
85 Second Street
San Francisco, California 94105

10 9 8 7 6 5 4 3 2 1

www.chroniclebooks.com

ACKNOWLEDGMENTS

This book is dedicated to all the women who shared their favorite cramp-kicking remedies with me. And to all the fellas out there baking the brownies and providing lower cone massages for their period-having pals.

Special Slurps-Up Milk Shake to the martial arts masters at Sockit Projects. Hot-outta-the-oven Red-Hot Brownies go to: Aunt Fran, D-Bros Tech Support, Dr. DeEtte DeVille, Alissa Faden, Ross Ginsberg, Bevin Lynch, Joanna Seitz, Julie McCue, Ashley Mullikan, Caitlin Nash, Marissa Perel C.F.R., Emily Rems, Bonnie Branson, Bridget Regan, Laura Barcella, Bilgin Turker, and Lenny Williams. Big thanks to the chocolate lovers at Chronicle Books: Mikyla Bruder, Alethea Morrison, Alicia Bergin, and Debra Lande. And thanks to my mom for teaching me how to pop wheelies on my BMX.

For more info about Vinnie: www.KNOWYOURFLOW.com
Or write to: vinnie@tamponcase.com

TABLE OF CONTENTS

VINNIE RX

 CRAMPS  PERIOD PAL   PMS 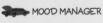 MOOD MANAGER

TENDER BOOBS   HEADACHES   BLOATING   BE PREPARED

VINNIE RX

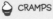

CRAMPS

TENDER BOOBS

PERIOD PAL

HEADACHES

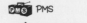 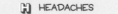

PMS

BLOATING

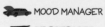

MOOD MANAGER

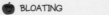

BE PREPARED

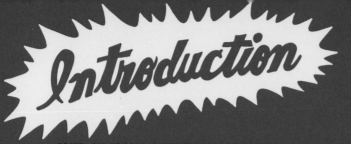

Introduction

ACNE. ALLERGIES. BOTHERSOME BROTHERS. OTHER GROSS BOYS. BRAS. BRACES. SPLIT ENDS. SISTERS. TUBE TOPS. WHITE JEANS. THE GLASS CEILING. ETC. BLECH.

With that list out of the way we can concentrate on the enjoyable stuff in life, like having your period. Yes, I know, enjoyment isn't the first emotion that comes to mind when you consider your monthly cycle—and it's probably not even the second emotion either—but this book is gonna change all that. Having crazy cramps or PMS or bloating will never be enjoyable, but the remedies I've packed into this book will at least make your efforts to reduce or eliminate them entertaining. So, enjoy yourself as you deliver a roundhouse kick to your cramps and a sucker punch to your PMS.

This book of cramp-kicking remedies is a compilation of cutting-edge cramp and PMS remedies culled from conversations with thousands upon thousands of Varsity and Junior Varsity menstruators. Since these remedies arrive tested and recommended by professional period-havers, there is a good chance you'll find a bunch that'll work for you.

Most of these reliable remedies can be easily implemented in and around your house (you might need a blender, some pretzel sticks, a sock, a soup can, and/or a cat). A bunch of these cramp-curing concepts involve the participation of a Period Pal (you know, someone sympathetic to your crazy cramps who has strong hands for massage and a speedy bike to go get you chocolate!).

I've taken the liberty to include not only remedies that reduce crazy cramps and sucker-punch PMS, but also a handful that deal with tender boobs, bloating, crankiness, and headaches. Who's looking out for you, right?

Since the monthly cycle is like your reliable mail carrier—ready to roll in rain, sleet, sun, or snow—I figured I'd group this book of remedies by season: spring, summer, fall, and winter. This will make it E-Z for you to reference the remedies throughout the year and make sure you are prepared no matter the weather. After all, cramps don't leave you to winter in West Palm Beach and PMS doesn't summer in Paris as part of a student exchange program, do they? So, think of this book as the all-weather gear for your period and PMS. Toss it in your beach bag or backpack, or strap it to your snowboard.

Take it wherever you go, and know the flow. —*Vinnie*

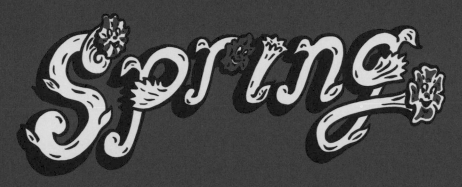

Springtime is hardly the season to be doubled over with cramps or extra-crabby with PMS. Love is in the air, flowers are blooming, your local ice-cream shop is opening for the season, and you have a new pair of white jeans ready for that special moment when your period surprises you at the weekend roller-skating party. (It's gonna happen—you might as well look the part. When it happens—act surprised.)

There are so many ways to relieve your cramps, it'll make your head spin. But, if you are already feeling kind of lousy with crazy cramps, who needs the head spins, too, right? Good point!

Read through these springy remedies and be ready to roll as soon as the groundhog sees her shadow (or when that cute kid from the laundromat finally gets up the nerve to ask you out for an Italian ice, whichever comes first).

THE BEST THINGS IN LIFE ARE FREE

The best things in life are free: sunsets, belly laughs, hand-me-down clothing, and library cards. And the best cramp remedies are also free: exercise and water. So do yourself a favor on a sunny spring day—grab your pals, a fistful of trail mix, and head for the hills. Breathe in that fresh clean air, pet a mountain goat, make a daisy necklace, return a wayward bald eagle chick to its nest atop a jagged cliff.

And while you are at it, don't forget to stay liquefied. It shouldn't be too hard to find fresh water at the source of a bubbling brook and gather a few gulps. Ahhh, tasty, pure spring water. Nothing quite like it. Crisp, clean, and cool. You'll barely miss the carbonation!

Water is vitally important to keeping your body hydrated and, amazingly, also keeps your cramps in check. Try drinking eight glasses throughout the day (or sixteen healthy gulps straight from the spring). Oh so easy, oh so free. You'll barely miss the cramps!

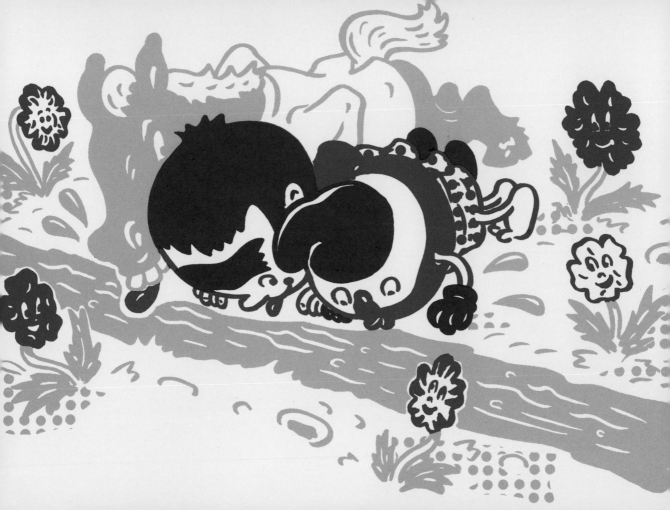

TWO-IN-ONE CRAMP-CRUNCH FOOT RUB

All this enthusiastic running barefoot through fields of flowers or running barefoot on the sidewalk to the ice-cream truck will take a toll on your feet. While your Period Pal is providing you with a friendly foot massage for your aching feet, sneak in a foot massage for your aching cramps! Believe it or not, there are points on your grass-stained feet that, when pressed correctly, will relieve your menstrual cramps. Whoa is right!

HERE'S HOW IT WORKS:
* Have your pal grab your right foot with their right hand, gently pressing their thumb in the space between your ankle and your heel and pressing their fingers in the same location on the other side of your foot.
* Then have them place the palm of their left hand against the ball of your foot.

You are now in position for "The Pump."
* Have your foot masseuse press forward with their left hand and pull your heel toward them with their right hand (see diagram A).
* Then have them place their left hand on the top of your foot and press forward while their right hand pushes the heel in (see diagram B).
* Do this flex 5 times, then switch feet and do another 5 pumps.

What could be better than a foot massage and a cramp massage at the same time? Maybe a foot massage and a cramp massage while you lie back and eat a Red-Hot Brownie (page 52).

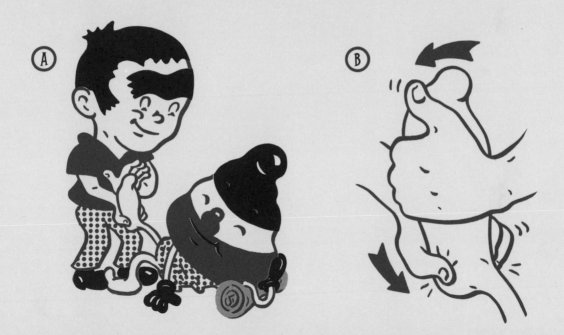

INSTANT REMEDY MESSAGING

It's sunny springtime and yet you find yourself moping through a cloudy case of PMS. There is no reason to be moping around feeling bad that your cramps have got you down when modern technology has made it nearly effortless to contact your pals the microsecond you feel that craving for chocolate or the nanosecond those crazy cramps twinge in your tummy. Don't waste a nano- or a microsecond! Hop on the e-mail or start tapping away on your instant-messaging device. Better yet, talk directly into your voice-activated wrist phone and alert your friends—no matter where they are—that you are in need of IMMEDIATE MENSTRUAL SUPPORT! Hopefully, your pals have already suspected that your period is on its way ('cause you gave 'em a period chart for their wallet and they've been counting the days since last month) and a batch of Red-Hot Brownies (page 52) are just about ready to come out of the oven. I can smell 'em from here.

REMEMBER: Keep your pals up to speed and they'll be there when you're in need.

JOG BRA DESCENDING THE STAIRCASE

Boobs.

Boobs hurt sometimes in the days before and sometimes during your period. Forget about volleyball practice!

My pal Dr. DeEtte DeVille says this has something to do with increased estrogen during your cycle. Whatever. The science isn't gonna save you from the discomfort as you rush to your next class, down two flights of stairs. Ouch.

This is where an elasticky but supportive sports bra can save the day and bolster your boobs. Sports bras are specifically designed for the extrasporty to be able to perform at their best while their boobs stay secure and close to the body. Thus, sports bras are perfect when you are experiencing tender boobs during your menstrual cycle and want to keep the bounce to a minimum. Strap on a sports bra, run up those stairs, and spike to your heart's delight in volleyball practice.

NOTE: An oversized sports bra is perfect for keeping your aquarium with pet octopus secure as you transport it to and from show-and-tell (banana peel not included).

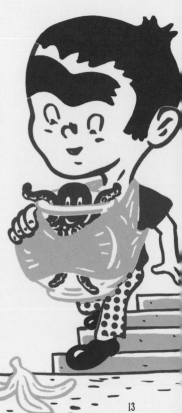

BURRITO LUMBAR-SUPPORT PILLOW

With all the springtime activity and excitement, you need to remember to keep your brain in motion, too. So grab your cramps and come inside for some popcorn and to finish reading the next chapter in your book. But, alas, trying to get comfortable on the couch and attempting to concentrate on your book is gonna be hard with your cramps going crazy.

This is a perfect time to create a Burrito Lumbar-Support Pillow. Amazingly, this well-placed support relieves your achy lower back by reconfiguring which muscles pick up the tab on keeping your back straight. You'll be amazed at how this simple creation will be able to assist you in combating your cramps in so many different ways.

YOU WILL NEED:
   1 hand towel   2 rubber bands
* Roll the hand towel up like a burrito and put a rubber band around each end.
* Prop the burrito pillow in the curve of your back between you and the couch.

This handy Burrito Pillow can be used in the car or in a regular chair as you study. There is no stopping the infinite uses of this bolstering burrito. It slices and dices cramps and makes mounds and mounds of coleslaw!

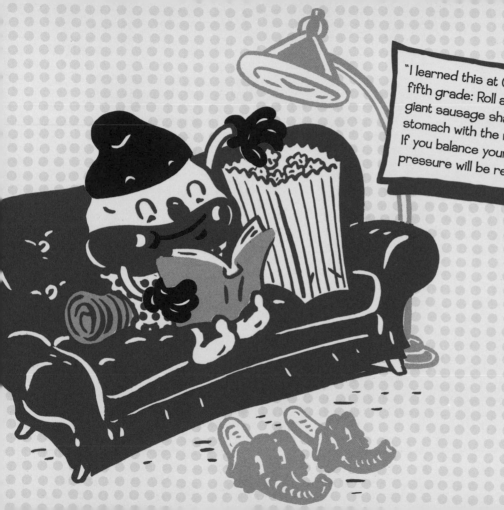

"I learned this at Girl Scout Camp in fifth grade: Roll a bath towel into a giant sausage shape and lay on your stomach with the roll under your hips. If you balance your pelvis just so, all pressure will be relieved." -LIBERTY

BURNIN' RUBBER BACK RUB

Everyone likes getting a back rub, but not everyone likes giving one. Not really fair, but what are you gonna do?

I recommend that instead of asking your Period Pal for a back rub, you ask to receive a BURNIN' RUBBER BACK RUB. You'll be surprised how this simple rewording will make the idea of giving a back massage that much more exciting!

The perfect lower-back massage is actually a lot like drag racing. Imagine that your spine is the drag strip. The bottom of your spine can be the starting point and right below your shoulder blades is the finish line. Ask your "driver" to pretend that each of their middle fingers is one of the big fat wheels on a dragster. Have your pal "burn rubber" with the "wheels" about two inches apart on either side of your spine.

Sounds like fun, huh! Remind your driver that the best dragsters have to go up and down the drag strip numerous times to get the feel of the track and to soften the wheels. Adjust the amount of burnt rubber to your personal taste.

It really helps the massage if your driver makes the sound of a dragster tearing up the track (these sounds will vary with each driver).

DRIVERS, START YOUR ENGINES! See you in the winner's circle (cramp free, of course).

CRAMP-CURIN' KIWI SHAKE

This all-natural, great-tasting cramp-curing drink is to cramp and crave for—and, amazingly, contains no chocolate! Fruits such as kiwis and bananas might actually be better for you than chocolate in terms of alleviating your cramps. Find out for yourself by trying the recipe below.

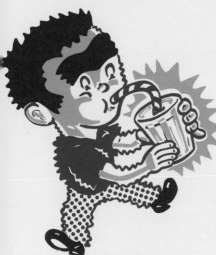

YOU WILL NEED:

1 medium banana, cut into 1-inch chunks

½ Granny Smith or other green apple, cut into 1-inch chunks

2 kiwis, peeled and quartered

½ cup enriched vanilla soy milk or cow's milk

4–5 ice cubes

* Toss all of these ingredients into the blender and watch 'em go round and round until you get a frothy lime-green milk-shake consistency.

* Pour into tall glasses and serve!

MAKES 2 SERVINGS

WARNING: Tartness will cause hair to stand on end and will get unwanted wrinkles out of polyester clothing.

EXERCISE ALTERNATIVE: BECOME A PRO WRESTLER

Running through fields of spring flowers or scraping the paint off of outdoor stair railings with your skateboard are primo ways to get exercise. Regular exercise keeps you in a good mood, gives you increased energy, and puts that rosy glow in your cheeks—and who doesn't like a rosy glow? Best of all, being fit makes your body less likely to experience the pain and discomfort of crazy cramps. But, since spring showers can call a halt to outdoor exercises, you might want to develop an indoor exercise backup.

How about wrestling? You can wrestle in the house—simply throw a few couch cushions on the floor of the living room and hire a manager. And if you get good at it, there is an entertaining and lucrative career waiting for you on the pro wrestling circuit (if you don't mind getting whapped in the head every once in a while with a folding chair).

Along with the obvious cardiovascular benefits to your year-round menstrual health, there are a few other important advantages to wrestling as a quality exercise option:

* You get to come up with a colorful name to intimidate your opponent.
* You can toss that obnoxious neighbor kid around the house.
* Maybe wrestle while you are experiencing PMS. What a great way to unleash your emotions!
* Your manager can screen your phone calls.

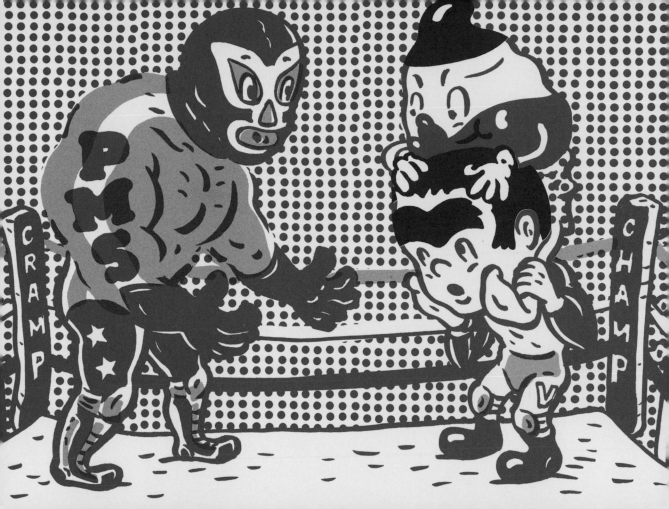

MIX-YOUR-OWN MINTY HEADACHE RELIEF RUB

Throwing around the annoying neighbor kid in your home-steel-cage-wrestling match (see page 18) is exhilarating, but the incessant screaming of the hundreds of fans packed into your living room sure can give you a headache.

So can your period.

Maybe it's time to calm down a tad.

Getting a horse to massage your tired temples with this excellent elixir of essential and aromatherapeutic oils is just what you need. A gentle temple massage with horse hooves (circular clockwise motions) combined with the pepperminty aromatherapy will tag-team most headaches.

Here's how to make your own relief rub. You can usually get all of these ingredients, except the horse, at a health-food store.

YOU WILL NEED:

    30 drops lavender essential oil

    20 drops peppermint essential oil

    Small bottle

    ½ ounce jojoba base oil or olive oil

       (for soft skin and great-tasting pasta!)

    Horse willing to apply the oil

* Combine the essential oils in the bottle; add the base
oil and swirl to blend.

* Have the horse rub the oil on your temples to relieve
headaches—be sure to avoid contact with your eyes.

* Reward the horse with sugar cubes, hay, or a pedicure.

MAKES ENOUGH RUB TO RELIEVE 100 HEADACHES

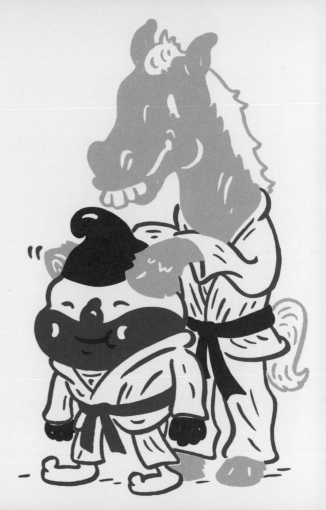

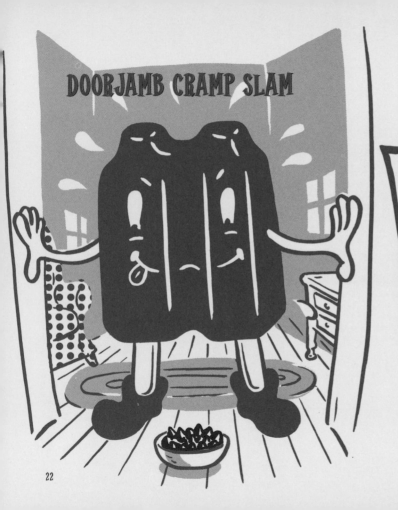

DOORJAMB CRAMP SLAM

"Hey Vinnie, my mom taught me to stand in a doorway and push with my arms on both sides of the doorjamb. Does that make sense? You are supposed to push real hard, and for some reason, VOILA! You have relief. Of course, if all else fails, chocolate chips always do the trick." -LORRE

SOUP-CAN SELF-MASSAGE

The best way to experience your monthly cycle is definitely with your pals—no need to go the flow alone. But, fact is, your pals aren't always around to make life exciting. In those moments when you find yourself on your own, you need to have a few backup remedies.

The Soup-Can Self-Massage is just the right remedy to keep in your waffle cone. All you need are a couple unopened cans of food. They don't have to be soup cans—in fact, my pal Emily, who revealed this remedy to me, says cans of spinach work best for no obvious scientific reason.

YOU WILL NEED:

  2 or more unopened cans of food

* Grab your cans and find a place on the floor where you can spread out. A rug is ideal so you don't scratch the floorboards. Place the cans on the floor on their side.
* Carefully lie down with your back on the cans (start with 2), placing one under your lower back and one near your shoulder blades.
* Using your feet to steer, slowly roll your body over the cans, gently rolling back and forth (see illustration).
* The desired effect should be similar to having a rubdown by the magical hands of an expert and ridiculously overpriced masseur. Okay, maybe not quite, but almost.

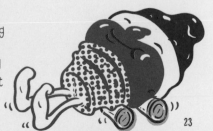

FLOP FORWARD YOGA POSE

The extra daylight that spring brings wreaks havoc on your internal clock. Before you know it, you have stuffed two days' worth of activity into one twenty-four hour period. Tiring. As you get fatigued, your cramps will be fatigued x 2. Cramps x 1 is enough—no need to double the trouble.

The Flop Forward Yoga Pose is a satisfying way to stretch out and relax to keep your cramps from multiplying.

YOU WILL NEED:
- A bolster—a couch cushion, a couple of pillows, or a few folded-up towels
- A box of doughnuts
* Kneel on the floor (kneeling on a rug will obviously be more comfortable than a hardwood floor).
* Spread your knees apart, but keep your toes touching.
* Put the bolster between your knees.
* Flop forward onto the bolster, exhaling as you go down.
* Flop your arms wherever they are comfortable.
* Make sure you are comfortable and rest in this position for 5–10 minutes.
* Eat a doughnut.

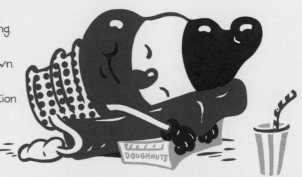

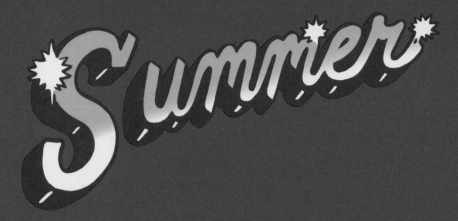

Summer is the easiest season for corralling your crazy cramps. Along with providing quality tannage, the sun is basically one gigantic cramp-melting device. All the heat it generates works to relax your muscles and soothe your cramps, whether you are lying out at the beach or serving ice cream at your summer job. For the sweltering summer, I've partnered up with the sun to provide you with a slew of satisfying solutions to keep you surfing with a smile all season long.

HOT ROCKS

Okay, so, you decide to go to the beach even though you aren't feeling your personal best. You can't stay home—especially since your pal's cute cousin from Calabria is also gonna be at the beach and who are you to pass up the opportunity to show off your Monster Truck bathing suit?

The Hot Rocks remedy is perfect when you are chillin' at the beach on a hot summer day. It works just like the dorky hot-water bottle your mom has under the bathroom sink except it's way less dorky, all natural, and can be applied at the beach! (For a clever way to un-dorkify your hot-water bottle, go to page 82.)

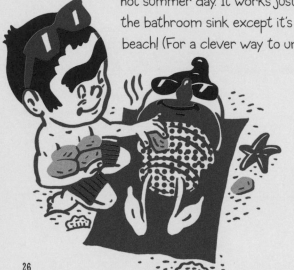

* Get a case of crazy cramps.
* Go to the beach with a bunch of your pals.
* Set out your beach blanket in the direction of the sun for primo tanning (after you've put on your sunscreen, of course!).
* Pull your supersize thermos of ice water out of your backpack and set down near your beach blanket (gotta stay hydrated).

* Walk around the beach and find a few flat rocks laying in the sand. By noon, rocks on the beach should be nice and hot (just like the sand under your feet). Grab a few flat rocks that are about the size of your hand and bring them back to your beach blanket.
* Put on your sunglasses, lie down, and place a few of the hot rocks on your stomach.
* Grab your favorite book and read away as the hot rocks melt those cramps.

Obviously, don't use rocks that are too hot—you can also put a shirt or a towel between your stomach and the hot rocks. And if you get too hot, just take a flying leap into the water.

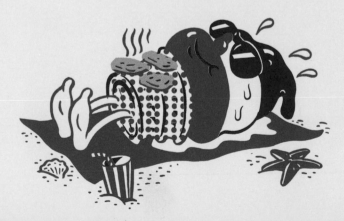

SUNBLOCK APPLICATION BACK RUB

OKAY, EVERYBODY FLIP!

After a good fifteen or twenty minutes with the hot rocks it's probably time to flip over—not for your tan! For your cramps! I've devised an ingenious way to eliminate your cramps while continuing to take full advantage of your beach day: the Sunblock Application Back Rub. Receiving a lower-back rub is probably the most popular cramp remedy—and having someone apply suntan lotion to your back is the next best thing.

YOU WILL NEED:

A volunteer   Plenty of sunblock

* Simply ask the lifeguard or your Period Pal if they would be kind enough to put some sunblock on your back—with an extra emphasis on your lower back.
* Advise the sunblock applier further that you tend to get sunburned on your lower back, so they really need to rub the sunblock in that area EXTRA firmly.

Who'd've thought you could soothe those cramps and protect yourself from harmful UV sun rays at the same time? Now you know.

BEACH BALL BUOYANCY BOOB RELIEVER

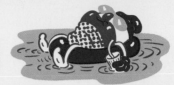

Tender boobs can be an uncomfortable booby prize of your monthly cycle. Even though it's funny to see the word BOOB in a book, tender boobs are not a laughing matter. They really can hurt and make it difficult to enjoy summertime fun. Luckily, there are ways to make your boobs feel better, even at the beach.

YOU WILL NEED:

A pool, an ocean, or a good-size lake

* Get in the water. If it's an ocean that you are getting into, you want to go beyond the waves (but, obviously, still within sight of the cute lifeguard); the last thing you want as part of this remedy is to be in rough waves. This is all about chilling out and floating in calm water. If you're at a pool, maybe wait until the kids are done splashing around before you jump in.
* Float on your back with your face toward the sun.
* Move your arms and legs just enough to keep yourself afloat. The water will surround you and support your boobs, allowing them to relax. Ahhh.

Even boobs deserve a buoyancy break every once in a while.

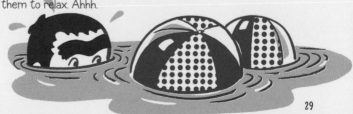

Being Zen About PMS Acne

It goes without saying that the monthly menstrual cycle is less fun than surfing. As if it weren't enough to deal with the PMS, cramps, and having to lug around all the gear related to your actual period, who needs acne on top of that? Acne on its own is enough of a drag. To have it brought on by your PMS, when you're already not feeling so chipper, is a double drag. I'm here to tell you that you can rise above the "drag" and ride the waves to a higher plane of inner utopia.

Okay, I can see your eyes rolling. Yeah, yeah—the last thing you need is Vinnie getting mystical on you. Don't worry—I'm not going there. All I'm saying is that there are things in this life you can control and there are things you can't control.

You can't always control PMS acne. No biggie. Follow the following directions for how to breathe through your blemishes. Save your anxiety for real issues like figuring out which side of the tube top goes to the front.

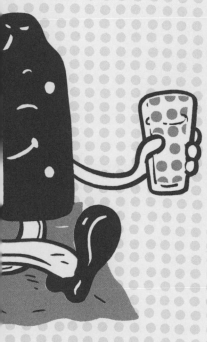

* Take 15 minutes out of your hectic schedule (you know, somewhere between karate practice and rock band practice), find a quiet spot, and sit down with your legs crossed.
* Close your eyes.
* Breathe in and out, preferably through your nose. (If you don't have a nose, breathe through your mouth.)
* Straighten your back (or sit up against a wall if you have an achy back).
* Keep breathing.
* Repeat after me:
    I really like brownies.
    I am one with my body.
    I will not let a few zits slow me down.
    I really like brownies.
* Repeat this simple chant until you feel better. Obviously, you should create a crazy-cramp karma chant that reflects your specific life—maybe you don't like brownies, maybe you like vanilla wafers instead, etc.
* Oh yeah—and drink a lot of water while you chant.

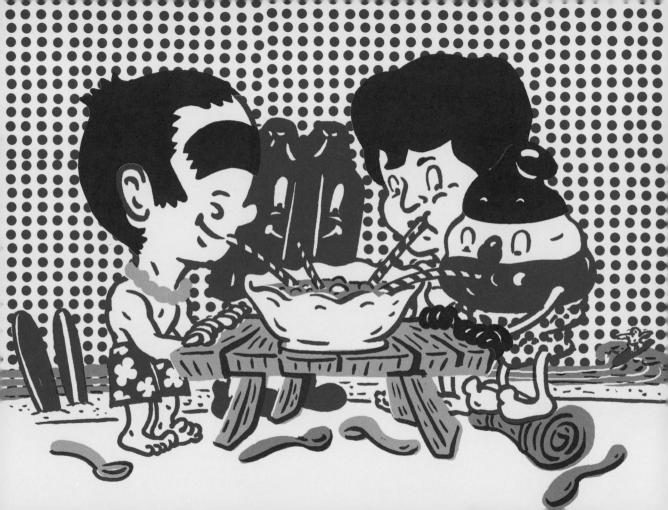

SLURPS-UP CALCIUM MILK SHAKE

DUDES! The Snack Shack at the beach that your older sis works at is more than a way to meet potential dates. It actually provides yet another rad way to keep a tanned leg up on your cramps. Turns out milk shakes are a great and tasty source of calcium. And calcium, when eaten four or so days before your period starts, can seriously reduce or eliminate your crazy cramps all together. It's the milk and ice cream in milk shakes that contain calcium, not the shake part. So, simply drinking plenty o' glasses of milk in the days before your period starts will do the trick as well.

But who wants a glass of milk at the beach when a frosty milk shake is on the menu? Here is the recipe for the Snack Shack's famous Slurps-Up Calcium Milk Shake.

YOU WILL NEED:

1/2 cup milk

1 cup blueberries

6 cups vanilla ice cream

20–24 drops blue food coloring

1 teaspoon vanilla

* Put all the ingredients in a blender and blend just until the shake is thick and yummy.
* Adjust the coloring 'til the shake is the color of the ocean.
* Slurps up!

MAKES 2 TO 3 SERVINGS

ESCAPE FROM SPINACH MOUNTAIN

Urban legend claims that the few who dared to scale Spinach Mountain never came back. The real story is that the few who dared did return—it was their cramps that never came back! **SPOOKY, EH?**

Like the Slurps-Up Milk Shake, spinach and other leafy greens are stuffed to the gills with calcium—the archenemy of cramps if eaten the week before your period starts. Follow the recipe below for a scarily good spinach salad.

YOU WILL NEED:

FOR THE SALAD

1 bunch spinach, washed, trimmed, and torn
    into bite-sized pieces
1/3 cup chopped walnuts
1/4 cup sunflower seeds
1/2 cup crumbled feta cheese
One 11-ounce can mandarin orange segments,
    drained, or peeled fresh orange segments

FOR THE DRESSING

1/4 cup freshly squeezed orange juice
3 tablespoons olive oil
1/4 teaspoon salt
Freshly ground pepper to taste
1 tablespoon balsamic vinegar

* Toss together the salad ingredients in your favorite salad bowl.
* To make the dressing, in a separate bowl, beat together the orange juice, olive oil, salt, and pepper using a fork or wire whisk.
* Add the vinegar and whisk to mix.
* Pour the dressing over the salad, toss, and serve immediately.

MAKES 4 ESCAPES

AND REMEMBER: The only way to escape from Spinach Mountain is to eat your way out!

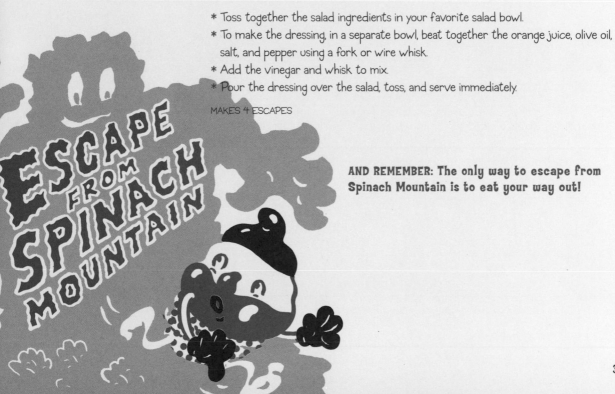

ESCAPE FROM SPINACH MOUNTAIN

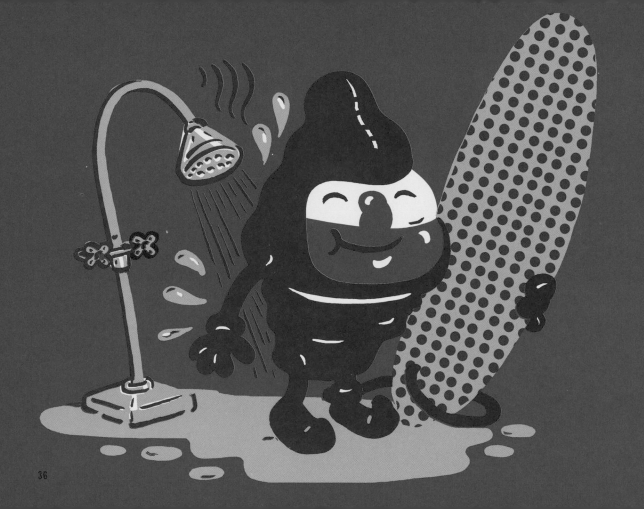

SATISFYING SURFER SHOWER

After a successful day at the beach you should be covered in sand, sun, and seaweed. Before you get on the subway to go home it'd be nice to wash off and maybe change out of your suit. Most beaches offer an outdoor shower for surfers to rinse off their boards and rinse the salt water out of their suits.

Often you'll see surfers standing and smiling under this cascade of hot water as it relieves their fatigued and achy muscles. A hot shower is a great way to relieve aches associated with menstrual cramps as well as aches associated with surfing. Hot water pulsating on your lower back serves as a gentle massage, and the heat will loosen up those cramping muscles. Ahhh.

Obviously, you can hit the showers at home no matter the season and direct that steady stream of water onto your lower back as a handy cramp cure.

SURF'S UP! CRAMPS DOWN!

SUMMERMINT SUN TEA

Tea just may be the most versatile cramp remedy of all. And when attempting to alleviate your cramps twelve times a year, versatility is a good thing. During the cold months, it's hard to beat the steamy cramp-curing goodness of a hot cup of tea. But once summer rolls around, it's hard to imagine sipping on a hot one in 100-degree heat.

This minty-cool combination of herbal tea and fresh mint puts a sleeperhold on your cramps and is so tasty you'll be craving it even in December. So whip up a batch and relax with your pals.

YOU WILL NEED:

2 tea bags of ginger tea

2 tea bags of red raspberry leaf tea

2 quarts of room-temperature water in a clear pitcher or jar, with lid

2 tablespoons honey

2 tablespoons fresh lemon juice

Ice

1 bunch of fresh mint

* Put all the tea bags in the pitcher of water and put on the lid.
* Set the pitcher in the sun for 3–6 hours until the tea is fully steeped.

* Add the 2 tablespoons of honey (or more if you like it sweeter) and
   2 tablespoons of lemon juice (or more if you like it more tart).
* Stir until the honey is completely dissolved.
* Add ice to your liking.
* Pour into tall tumblers.
* Add a couple sprigs of mint per glass.
* **ENJOY!**

MAKES 6 TO 8 SERVINGS

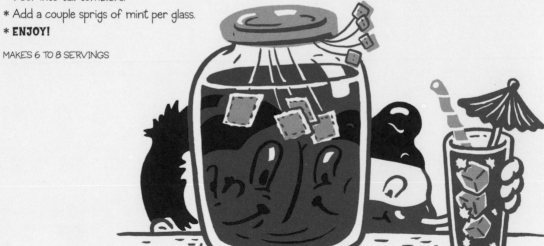

TAKE YOUR FLOW ON THE ROAD

It's one thing to have your remedies on hand around the house. It's quite another thing to be equipped to combat your cramps on the road. As they say: "Better safe than crampy."

So, when the station wagon is getting loaded up for the family road trip, be sure to pack along all your favorite remedies. If you have been charting your period (for charting info see page 86), you'll have an idea when on the trip you can expect tender boobs (Yellowstone), PMS (Grand Canyon to the Redwood Forests), or crazy cramps (Vegas).

Of course, most vacation destination points will offer access to remedies, including ones you may not have tried yet (hot springs in Palm Desert, California, or a Jacuzzi at a roadside hotel), but it's best to bring along a few standbys.

Here are a few remedies that are E-Z to pack and will help out in a pinch:

* Mix-Your-Own Minty Headache Relief Rub (page 20)
* Burrito Lumbar-Support Pillow (page 14)
* Comfy Chamo Tea (page 62) or All-Mixed-Up Tea (page 81)
* This book (so you have correct massage techniques and other quick tips at hand)

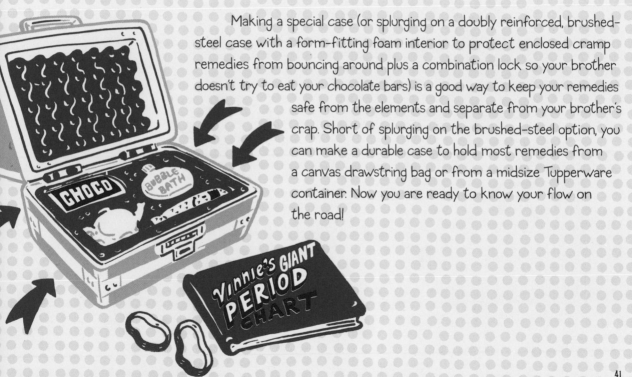

Making a special case (or splurging on a doubly reinforced, brushed-steel case with a form-fitting foam interior to protect enclosed cramp remedies from bouncing around plus a combination lock so your brother doesn't try to eat your chocolate bars) is a good way to keep your remedies safe from the elements and separate from your brother's crap. Short of splurging on the brushed-steel option, you can make a durable case to hold most remedies from a canvas drawstring bag or from a midsize Tupperware container. Now you are ready to know your flow on the road!

FUGIDABOUDIT PMS HEADACHE FOOT RUB

Every summer I help my grandmother tie off her tomato plants with the elastic from recycled bras. Really. I admit it's kind of funny, but you can't knock her clever recycling instinct and, heck, she grows the best tomatoes.

My grandmother was born in a small town in the hills of Sicily, Italy. When she was twenty-seven she moved to New York City. Even though she didn't speak English when she got to New York, she speaks it pretty fluently now. One of her favorite words in English is "fugidaboudit." This is actually the phrase "forget about it" smushed together like a peanut butter cookie and pretzel stick sandwich (page 80).

If you ask her if anyone makes a better meatball, she'll say, "Fugidaboudit."

If you ask her if there was ever a better singer than Dean Martin, she'll also say, "Fugidaboudit."

If you ask her for a great way to relieve a PMS headache, she'll say, "Try the Fugidaboudit Foot Rub."

And she's right. Anyone who knows anything about reflexology (the art of massaging points in your feet to help relieve other parts of your body) knows that rubbing your toes the right way can reduce a headache in heartbeat.

The toes are the head reflex. That didn't mean anything to me until my pal Marissa, a pro toe reflexologist, showed me how it works. If you have a headache, get Marissa or a pal with dexterous fingers to perform the following on your toes (maybe do them a favor and wash your feet first). Have your personal reflexologist follow these steps as you lie back and relax:

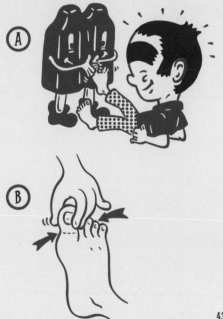

TOE ROLL
* Roll the toes between your hands (see diagram A). Gently roll-massage each toe starting, with the big toe.

TOE TUMBLE
* Gently move each toe around in a circular motion.

GEAR SHIFT
* Place the edge of your thumb firmly against the outside of the toe and grip the inside of the toe with your fingers. Bend each toe back and forth (see diagram B).

TOE TRACE
* Massage the whole surface of the bottom of each big toe with your thumb. Go around and around in a counter-clockwise circle.

KNOW YOUR TOES AND YOUR FLOW.

BEND A WRESTLER'S EAR

No matter whether your PMS or cramps tag along on your summer va-cay to the Grand Canyon or whether they join you at your summer job in town, it's important to have someone you can complain to about the pain. If you can't think of anyone off the top of your head, I have a suggestion: pro wrestlers.

Pro wrestlers are accustomed to pain. They get tossed around, stepped on, kicked, elbowed, hit with folding chairs, and sometimes even tossed right out of the ring and onto a cement floor **OUCH.** They know pain. As a result, they are great to consult with if you are experiencing crazy cramps. They know what it's like to be doubled over in agony and probably have a few pointers on how to make you feel better.

Pro wrestlers are also great to share your concerns regarding PMS with. The mood swings of PMS are not unlike the personality switch a wrestler goes through in and out of the wrestling ring. In the ring, wrestlers are short-tempered, stubborn, and emotional (sound familiar?). Outside of the ring, they are more or less normal. Since their profession requires this exaggerated personality transition they can COMPLETELY relate to the exaggerated mood swings of PMS.

So, I recommend talking to pro wrestlers if you are having a tuff time with PMS or cramps and need a sympathetic ear.

If you don't have a pro wrestler readily available, I recommend finding someone else to share your concerns with. No reason to keep your frustration to yourself, and there are tons of folks (over HALF the population of the world! Around three billion people!) who, like pro wrestlers, know exactly what you are going through.

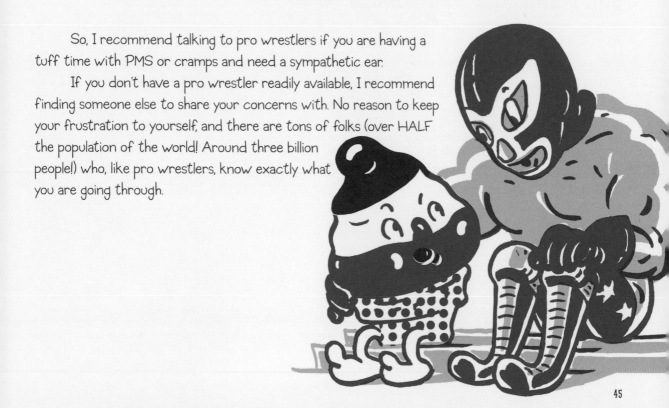

HOT VINNASANA

Once you are home from a hectic day at the beach and before you rush out to go to the movies, you might need to take a couple minutes to chill out. The Hot Vinnasana is a valuable (and easy!) yoga pose that is perfect for recharging your system and for soothing your cramps.

I know this picture looks like Hot Vinn is sleeping and not doing anything yoga-ish. But he is. This is the Hot Vinnasana yoga pose. The idea with this pose is to lie on your back with your arms out at your sides, palms up, and completely relax your body for ten or so minutes.

A couple ways to add to the relaxation is to use an eye pillow (see the Extra-Thick Aromatherapy Eyebrow Pillow on page 68) or to put a soft support under your knees (such as the Burrito Lumbar-Support Pillow on page 14).

Taking ten minutes out of your busy schedule to chill during your period is important and A-OK.

* Lie down in a comfortable spot on the floor.
* Place a Burrito Pillow or other soft support under your knees.
* Place an eye pillow over your eyes.
* Keep your legs shoulder-width apart and your feet relaxingly flopped to the sides.
* Rest your arms comfortably several inches from your sides, with the palms of your hands up.
* Relax your limbs; relax your neck and shoulders.
* Be sure to breathe through your nose.
* Stay in this position for *10–15* minutes, or until your cat comes and sits on your stomach.

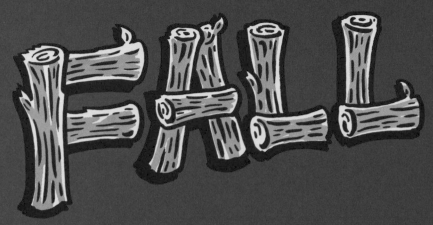

Your cramps are back after being in Paris all summer as part of the Cramp Exchange Program. At least it feels like you had the summer off from your cramps—thanks to the amount of time you spent at the beach letting the sun melt your cramps away. But now it's fall—your tan is fading, the sand is out of your shoes, and your cramps are oddly craving a chocolate croissant. Go get the croissant, grab a sweater, sit at a café with this book, and begin committing to memory the following fully functional fall remedies.

MOBILE BACKACHE-RELIEVING MACHINE

If only you could program your cramps like you can program the VCR to tape your favorite TV show to watch later. Then you would simply program your cramps to happen for the least intrusive part of your day—and you'd be sure to be ready for 'em with all your favorite remedies. Heck, if you could program 'em you'd just program them not to happen at all, right?

Unfortunately, cramps can happen at any part of the day—whether you are at home and ready for 'em or whether you are out and about making the most of your day. And when you are out, with your backpack over your shoulders, the last thing you need slowing you down is lower-back aches from your crazy cramps.

Here's a way to put the kibosh on your cramps even as you cruise through your daily commute—my Mobile Backache-Relieving Machine.

Stuff your hot-water bottle into your Hot Vinn Custom Water-Bottle Cozy, slide it snugly into the bottom of your backpack (between you and your books), and feel the portable heat banish your backache to oblivion.

YOU WILL NEED:

Hot-water bottle

Hot Vinn Custom Water-Bottle Cozy (page 82)

Comfy backpack

* Go to sleep.
* Wake up about 8 hours later.
* Slowly scarf down your breakfast.
* Fill your hot-water bottle with hot water. Screw on the cap nice and tight.
* Insert the hot-water bottle inside your Hot Vinn Custom Water-Bottle Cozy and then plop this inside your backpack. Feel the heat as you strut down the street!

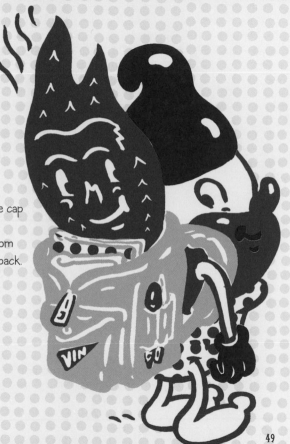

CLASS-IC LOWER CONE MASSAGE

As much as you'd like to send your cramps to the proverbial principal's office while you concentrate on life's lessons, you can't. These crazy cramps deserve an A for effort, but you need to flunk 'em anyway. So, at the privacy of your own desk, take a short break and have a pal provide you with the Lower Cone Massage.

HERE'S HOW YOU DO IT:

* Clear your desk of all detritus.
* Lean forward and put your head down on your desktop.
* Find an assistant with strong fingers (hint: any pal with speedy keyboard skillz probably has dexterous digits!).
* Have your assistant use both thumbs to give you a quick but high-quality lower cone massage:
    1. Rub the thumbs along either side of the ice-cream cone's spine about 1 1/2 inches from the spine's ridge. About 4 inches above the bottom of the cone (or the top of your butt) is the perfect spot to begin.
    2. Rub the thumbs in clockwise circles or up and down along either side of the spine (like the Burnin' Rubber Back Rub, page 16).
* Erase your cramps, get back to the head of the class, and reward yourself and your masseuse with a brownie.

GLAZED DOUGHNASANA

When you are doubled over with a case of crazy cramps, you might think the gym is the last thing you need—you're definitely not in a synchronized swimming mood, and the only weights you feel like lifting are a few chocolate milk shakes. On the other hand, changing into comfortable gym clothes to stretch in a less hectic corner of the gym could be just what you need.

So, use the gym to your advantage and do this simple yoga pose designed specially to relieve your cramps. With an intriguing Sanskrit name like "The Glazed Doughnasana," you'd be crazy not to give it a try.

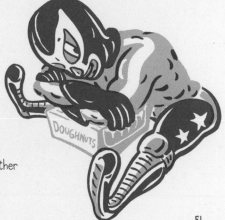

HERE'S HOW TO DO THE GLAZED DOUGHNASANA:
* Sit on the floor.
* Stretch your legs into a comfortable, wide V.
* Cross your arms in front of you and lean forward onto a box of doughnuts (or any similar support device; a rolled-up mat if you are in the gym or a couple couch pillows if you are at home).
* Your head and neck should be in line with your spine.
* Hold this position for 5 minutes.
* You should feel comfortable resting on the doughnut box or pillows, rather than feeling overly stretched out.
* Eat a doughnut.

AUNT FRAN'S RED-HOT BROWNIES

If you've been suffering through a whole day of cramps, you need a reward. Why not swing by Aunt Fran's Red-Hot Brownie Truck on the way home?

The most important thing you can do for your body is listen to it. If your body is craving chocolate, maybe you need to have a GIANT Red-Hot Brownie—or five GIANT Red-Hot Brownies!

And if it's a GIANT Red-Hot Brownie you crave, then my Aunt Fran's world-famous Red-Hot Brownie recipe is the one to reach for—they are E-Z to make and E-Z-er to eat!

YOU WILL NEED:

4 ounces unsweetened baking chocolate
3/4 cup butter
1 cup flour
1 teaspoon baking powder
1/4 teaspoon salt

1 1/2 cups sugar
3 eggs
1 teaspoon vanilla
1 cup semisweet chocolate chips
1/2 cup Red Hots

* Preheat the oven to 350 degrees F.
* Lightly butter a 9-by-13-inch baking pan and line the bottom of the pan with parchment paper.
* Melt the baking chocolate and butter together in a double boiler or microwave, stirring occasionally, then set aside to cool.

* Sift together the flour, baking powder, and salt in a small bowl.
* Pour the cooled chocolate mixture into a large bowl.
* Gradually add the sugar to the chocolate mixture while stirring.
* Beat the eggs and vanilla into the chocolate mixture.
* Fold the flour mixture into the chocolate mixture, then fold in the chocolate chips and two-thirds of the Red Hots.
* Spread the batter evenly in the prepared pan.
* Sprinkle the remaining Red Hots on top.
* Bake for 30 minutes, or until done (you know they're done when a toothpick stuck in the middle of the brownies comes out clean).
* Let cool 1 hour before cutting.

MAKES 12 TO 15 BROWNIES, ENOUGH TO SHARE WITH A FEW FRIENDS OR EAT ON YOUR OWN ALL AT ONCE!

PUMPKIN SEED SNACK

I'll bet you didn't know that jack-o'-lanterns were originally created to hang in windows to ward off PMS. Okay, I made that up. But pumpkins can help you ward off another period predicament: Turns out that pumpkin seeds are the perfect pacifier for bloating. That's right, I said BLOATING. As your period starts, you retain water (can you tell I'm reading right out of a health manual or what!). This water retention expands your belly and makes you feel weighted down and less than fabulous. Eating fibrous foods, such as vegetables and fruits, and eating foods high in magnesium, like nuts and pumpkin seeds, the week before your period starts will greatly reduce the possibility of bloating. **BRING ON THE PUMPKIN SEEDS!**

Once you've carved out your pumpkin with a really scary face, dry out the pumpkin seeds and serve 'em up. Makes for a perfect snackable instead of popcorn as you watch a movie with your pals.

YOU WILL NEED:

Large pumpkin

Knife

Big spoon or hand

Colander or bowl

2 tablespoons olive oil

Baking sheet

Votive candle

Salt

Cut off the top of the pumpkin and save the top as a lid.

Scoop out the seedy stringy interior and put it in the colander or bowl.

Pull all the stringy pumpkin off the seeds.

Rinse the seeds and let them dry.

Preheat the oven to 350 degrees F.

Drizzle the olive oil on the seeds and stir them so they're coated.

Spread the seeds on the baking sheet and bake for 30 minutes, or until lightly browned.

Meanwhile, carve a giant eyebrow into the pumpkin insert a candle, light it, and pop the lid on your new Vinn-o'-lantern.

Toss the toasted seeds with salt and enjoy!

MAKES 1 VINN-O'-LANTERN AND A LOOT-BAG FULL OF PUMPKINS SEEDS.

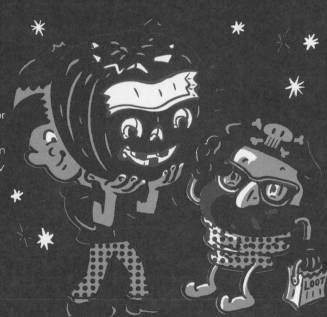

PERSONALIZE YOUR PMS IRON-ON T-SHIRTS

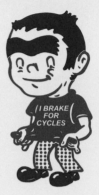

Remember when you sprained your ankle skateboarding? It wasn't that big a deal, you iced it for twenty minutes and had a slight limp at school the next day. Remember all the attention you got for that limp? Cute classmates holding doors, an extra scoop of mac-n-cheese from the lunch lady, not having to take out the garbage at home…it really wasn't THAT big a deal but everyone was so willing to go out of their way to make your life a tad easier.

Why doesn't this happen when you are doubled over with really bad cramps? Or when you are extremely sensitive and emotional due to PMS? Well, Vinnie's here to tell you why: It's because nobody knows when you have PMS or bad cramps, because it's not as obvious as a limp from a sprained ankle. To combat this lack of deserved attention for your monthly cycle, I've come up with a solution: Personalized PMS T-Shirts.

Put your favorite PMS (or period-related) phrase front and center for everyone to read. All you need is a T-shirt and some iron-on letters—It's E-Z, and everyone will now know the flow. May the extra brownies begin (every month)!

YOU WILL NEED:

   T-shirt

   Iron-on letters (found at your local fabric store)

   Iron

   Creative inspiration

* Ponder your period. What message will gain you the most support for your cycle?
Here are a few ideas from the Vinnster:

   FEED ME CHOCOLATE The truth always makes for a good slogan.

   I BRAKE FOR CYCLES A clever twist on an old favorite.

   PMS IS NOT A CRIME PMS needs support, not a parking ticket.

   KNOW THE FLOW A catchy reminder to guys and gals to do the right thing.

* Lay out your iron-on letters on your shirt to make sure they fit.

* Place your shirt on an ironing board or a folded-over towel on a table.

* Iron your letters in place.

* Let your shirt cool.

* Put on your shirt and break up the monotony in other people's days.

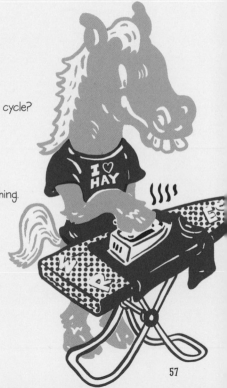

RATE YOUR DATE

What's worse than having really crazy cramps the same day you are supposed to go on a date with that cute ice-cream scooper from your fave ice-cream shop? I'll tell you what's worse—if the ice-cream scooper shows no sympathy for your pesky period predicament. Having cramps or PMS turns out to be a great way to rate your date. Last thing you want is to be with somebody that has no sympathy for your discomfort.

Even better than sympathy is a date who might come equipped to make you feel better—i.e., chocolates, extra-bubbly bubble bath, homemade peanut butter cookie and pretzel stick sandwiches (page 80), a Vinnie's Tampon Case (page 60), a funny movie rental (page 65), etc....

Expecting a date to be cramp conscious is the correct expectation, but you should be prepared in case the date turns out to be a dud. Maybe even save yourself the hassle of putting on your best pair of jeans and those fake eyelashes. A simple phone call to your date with a few choice questions will make it crystal clear whether this date is worthy of your valuable time.

SAMPLE MULTIPLE-CHOICE QUESTIONS TO HELP RATE BEFORE YOU DATE:

* A woman has her period approximately every:
    a. day
    b. month
    c. year
    d. time it rains

* During their cycle many women crave:
    a. chocolate
    b. asparagus
    c. castor oil

* Menstrual cramps can be relieved by:
    a. whistling a happy tune
    b. filling out the appropriate forms
    c. taking a relaxing, hot bubble bath

* If a woman is experiencing PMS, you can support her by:
    a. running the other direction
    b. pretending she is simply crazy
    c. offering her a soothing foot massage

* If you want to really make a good impression on a first date, you can:
    a. brush your teeth first
    b. show up with a pint of chocolate ice cream
    c. not judge someone if they eat all the ice cream at once
    d. all of the above

CRAMP-AND-TAMP TOTE— MAKE YOUR OWN VINNIE'S TAMPON CASE

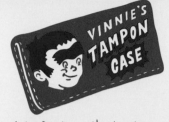

Whether you are going on a date or on a field trip to the chocolate factory, the best way to be prepared for your monthly cycle's multifaceted needs is to have a variety of cycling accoutrements on hand when you leave the house.

The best container for this is, obviously, my Vinnie's Tampon Case—a durable cramp-and-tamp carryall protecting period products in all the coolest backpacks, pockets, and purses. Get yourself an original Vinnie's Tampon Case or make your own.

Here are directions for making a simple yet fully functional cramp/tamp tote that is sturdy enough to keep your period products from getting broken at the bottom of your bag.

YOU WILL NEED:
- One sheet of 14-by-8 inch sturdy paper (card stock)
- Colored permanent pens
- Sturdy tape (fabric tape, movie gaffer's tape)
* Design the image for decorating your case. (Draw by hand or fashion a layout on a computer.)

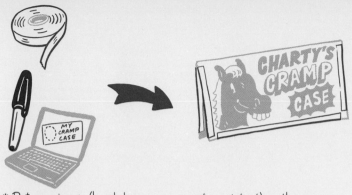

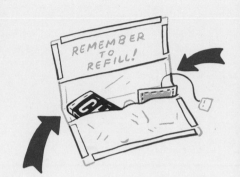

* Put your image (hand drawn or computer printout) on the paper
* Lay the paper, image-side down, on the table.
* Fold over ½ inch of the top and bottom edges of the paper.
* Fold over ½ inch of the side edges of the paper.
* Fold the whole piece of paper in half so it makes a 6½-by-7-inch rectangle.
* Open the paper back up and lay it flat. Using the crease of the center fold as a guide, fold each half of the paper toward the center fold, like you're closing the shutters on a window, leaving a ½-inch gap between each edge and the center fold. Line the edges up straight and press to crease.
* Affix tape along the side edges to create the internal pockets.
* Stuff with all your period gear and hit the road!

NOTE: If you want to make a fabric case, simply subsitute sturdy fabric for the paper and sew up the seams instead of taping them.

COMFY CHAMO TEA

When you are home for the night and settling in to practice a few handstands while doing a crossword puzzle, it is easy to get distracted. Heck, between the phone ringing and your loud wanna-be opera-singer neighbor, it's amazing you can concentrate at all. But you don't rock the crossword section every week by giving in to distraction. Ignoring the phone, tuning out the warbly singing, and maintaining the handstand is the only way to focus on a nine-letter cramp cure that is also an aromatic perennial herb native to Europe and the Mediterranean region.

You also know that when your cramps are going crazy, you have to take a moment or two to buckle down and focus on relieving them with the same determination you give the crossword puzzle. So, if you can get out of the handstand and put down your Number 2 pencil for fifteen or twenty minutes to brew a pot of soothing chamomile tea, then do it. No need to power through your crampy discomfort when relief is conveniently behind a cupboard.

YOU WILL NEED:

1 chamomile tea bag   Honey to taste

* Bring a teakettle of water to a boil.
* Drop the tea bag into a mug of the hot water.
* Add a tad of honey (optional yet tasty).

* Turn off your cell phone.
* Turn off the overhead lights.
* Turn off your anxiety.
* Put your feet up.
* Sip your tea.
* Turn off your cramps.

A study break with a cup of chamomile tea, a comfy chair, and a pair of closed eyes is a classic cramp-cure combination.

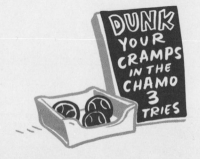

DUNK
YOUR
CRAMPS
IN THE
CHAMO
3
TRIES

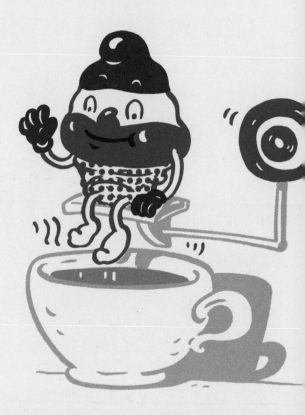

SOOTHING BUBBLE BEATS AND BOOMIN' BASS

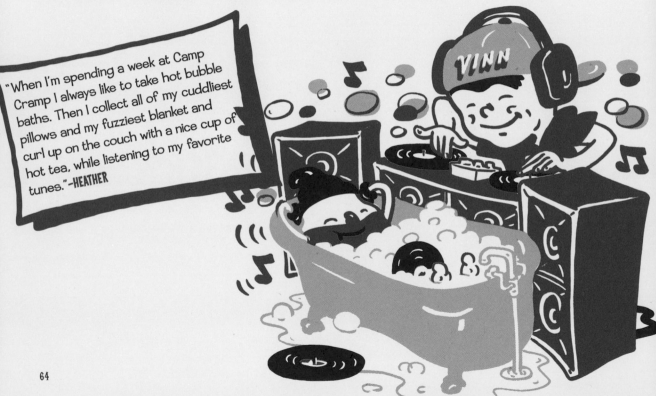

"When I'm spending a week at Camp Cramp I always like to take hot bubble baths. Then I collect all of my cuddliest pillows and my fuzziest blanket and curl up on the couch with a nice cup of hot tea, while listening to my favorite tunes." –HEATHER

CRANKY CURE-ALL

Let's face it—nobody wants to be cranky. But, fact is, when you are dealing with the mood swings or cramps from your period it's hard to keep that smile lighting up Broadway 24-7. We're human after all—and when humans turn cranky there's nothing better than climbing under a blanket with the remote in hand (and maybe a bowl of ice cream in the other...) and clicking on your favorite funny movie rental.

I'm here to tell you that there is nothing wrong with tuning out your discomfort and tuning in your favorite laff riot. Heck, every scientist knows that a good belly laugh cures everything—especially cramps. So, get your pals to come over (optional but recommended) and laugh your crankiness away.

* Rent funny movie (maybe get one you've seen before to guarantee a healthy chuckle).
* Drag warm blanket to couch in living room or drag the TV to bedroom.
* Climb under blanket.
* Watch funny movie.
* Laugh.
* Repeat.

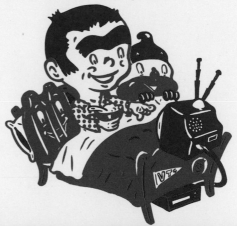

TAKE YOUR CRAMPS TO THE CLEANERS

Another cool way to bring the heat to your cramps in the comfort of your home is by trans-forming the bathroom into a spa-style steam room. Steam heat is like bringing your cramps to the dry cleaners—smoothes out the rough edges and provides same-day service. So steam up the bathroom, sit back, and steam clean your cramp's clocks.

YOU WILL NEED:

Bathrobe   Refreshing drink in a tall glass (try Summermint Tea, page 38)
A pair of flip flops   Comfortable wooden chair

* Put on the robe and flip flops.
* Have your drink within reach of your spa spot.
* Bring the wooden chair into your bathroom.
* Turn the shower on to high heat.
* Sit back in the wooden chair, close your eyes, and breathe deeply.
* Fifteen minutes of this moist steam heat will do wonders to relax
  and relieve your cramps.

Also, if you are dealing with PMS, it's hard to beat a soothing steam-room meditation, com-plete with the soothing sounds of a babbling brook (okay, really the sound of the water hitting the shower curtain—but we're using our imaginations right?).

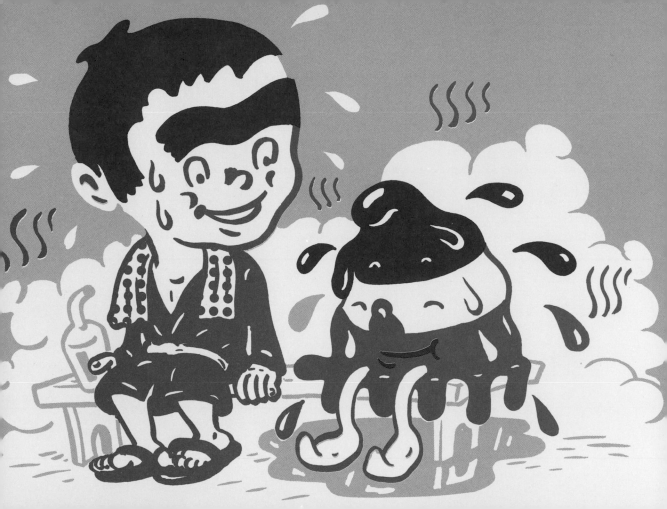

EXTRA-THICK AROMATHERAPY EYEBROW PILLOW

Smells are a powerful thing. All I need is one whiff of my Grandma Joya's spaghetti sauce and I can be happy for days. Now THAT'S aromatherapy!

This same aromatherapy concept can be put to work relieving your cramps by using my Extra-Thick Aromatherapy Eyebrow Pillow. Even if the pillow is designed to look like my giant eyebrow, the general idea here is to provide gentle, relaxing pressure on your eyeballs and soothing aromatherapy for your cramps. This is YOUR Extra-Thick Aromatherapy Eyebrow Pillow, so feel free to customize the filler as you see fit. You can substitute Red-Hots for the flaxseed, rose petals or fresh-cut lawn grass for the scented herbs, etc.

YOU WILL NEED:
Two 9½-by-4½-inch pieces of black felt
Needle and thread
2 tablespoons dried rosemary or lavender (both of these soothing
    smells are easily procured from most health-food stores)
1½–2 cups flaxseed (also readily available at health-food stores)

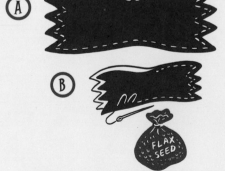

* Line up one piece of felt over the other and cut out a shape that looks like my eyebrow (see diagram A).
* Starting $\frac{1}{8}$ inch from the edge, sew around the eyebrow shape until you get about $2\frac{1}{2}$ inches from where you started (see diagram B).
* You now have a nearly completed sewn eyebrow with a small hole to pour in your aromatherapy filler.
* Mix your choice of scented herb with the flaxseed, pour into your felt eyebrow, and then finish sewing it up.
* Lie back and set the eyebrow pillow over your eyes.
* Relax as the double eyebrow sends your cramps over the rainbow.

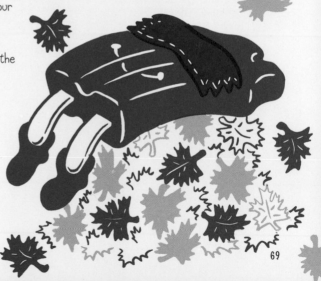

TOFU BOO COOKIES

I'm sure for a bunch of you out there the idea of eating tofu is scarier than most Halloween costumes. Don't be scared. Tofu is your friend. The same way a potato is your friend once it is chopped up, deep-fried, slathered with salt and ketchup, and called a French fry. And what a good friend the potato has turned out to be!

Uncooked tofu tastes just like a potato without any fixings—pretty bland. But as it turns into a tasty Halloween dinner treat called the Tofu Boo Cookie, I'm certain you'll become fast friends. And, better yet, unlike your pal the potato, your new pal tofu is a great source of calcium—the cool new way to eliminate your cramps before they get started. Word around town is that eating a boat-load of calcium four days before your period starts can scare the cramps right outta your body.

YOU WILL NEED:

¼ cup soy sauce

5 tablespoons olive oil

¼ teaspoon dried rosemary

2 tablespoons fresh basil, chopped

Freshly ground pepper to taste

¼ cup balsamic vinegar

2 cloves garlic, finely chopped

2 teaspoons ground turmeric

1 tablespoon honey

Two 1-pound blocks of extra-firm tofu

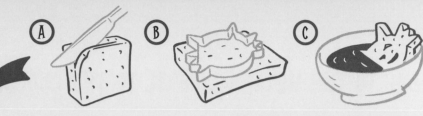

(A)   (B)   (C)

* Mix the soy sauce, 3 tablespoons olive oil, rosemary, basil, pepper, vinegar, garlic, turmeric, and honey together in a baking dish; be sure to stir until the honey is fully dissolved.
* Slice each block of tofu lengthwise into 4 slabs, each about ½ inch thick.
* Cut each slab in a kooky cookie shape using your favorite cookie cutters.
* Place the tofu shapes in the marinade, making sure that they are covered with the liquid.
* Marinate for as long as you have time, at least 30 minutes and up to overnight.
* Preheat the oven to 375 degrees F.
* Spread the remaining 2 tablespoons olive oil around on a rimmed baking sheet.
* Carefully drain the marinated tofu pieces, then place on the oiled pan and turn once to coat. Discard the marinade.
* Bake for 15 minutes. Flip the tofu cookies carefully with a spatula and cook for 15 minutes longer, for a total of 30 minutes.
* Remove from the oven and serve! These taste great with Escape from Spinach Mountain (page 34).

MAKES 4 SERVINGS

PEDAL TO THE METAL VS. PEDAL TO THE CHOCOLATE

You don't need a person with an oversized eyebrow to remind you that keeping your body in shape is maybe the best cramp cure of 'em all, but I'm gonna tell you anyway. Riding your bike a couple days a week is a hella swella way of shakin' your bacon and keeping your body loose and limber. Crazy cramps and moody PMS steer clear of helmet wearers. I don't know why, they just do.

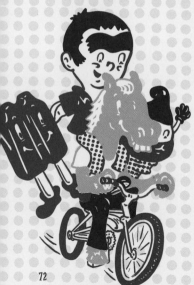

Where you trek on your bike is completely up to you. You may decide to ride your bike to the local ice-cream parlor to get a scoop or you may decide to simply ride around your neighborhood, pick up all your friends on the same bike, and become some kind of kooky bike-riding circus act. Be careful going down steep hills like this or riding near low-hanging tree branches.

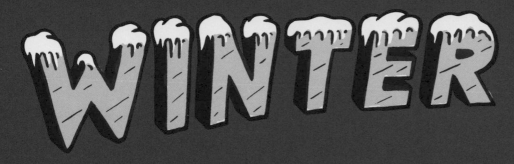

WINTER

Winter is frozen solid with cool ways to keep your cramps and PMS on ice. Example #1: chestnuts.

Chestnuts roasting over an open fire is a tradition of winter. I'll bet if you grabbed a handful of hot chestnuts, tossed 'em in a paper bag, and placed the bag on your tummy, you could create your own cramp-curing winter tradition. I'm telling you, cramp-curing is E-Z if you are able to think outside of the igloo.

So take advantage of the wonderland with remedies like the Hot Vinn Deluxe and the Hot Cocoa Kebob—you'll be toasty all season long and your cramps will be left out in the cold.

HOT SPRINGS ETERNAL

With the sun up for only a handful of hours, getting heat to your achy and crampy back muscles is the trick in the winter. Not always easy, unless you conveniently live next to natural hot springs. These wonders of nature, piping-hot water bubbling out of the ground like a Jacuzzi volcano, will work wonders for your cramps. Natural hot springs run all year-round, and stay hot even in cold weather.

YOU WILL NEED:

Snowshoes (optional)   Thermos of hot cocoa (page 76)

* Snowshoe or hike with your pals to the closest hot springs and hop in.
* Say "yes" if the abominable snowman asks to join you.
* Pass around the thermos of hot cocoa.
* Enjoy the bubbling hot water melting your cramps.

HOME HOT SPRINGS VARIATION: Not everyone lives near natural hot springs, but there are ways to re-create the experience at home.

* Turn off the heat in your house (optional).
* Fill the tub with hot water.
* Put the cocoa in a mug and get in the tub.
* Enjoy the hot water and hot cocoa melting your cramps.

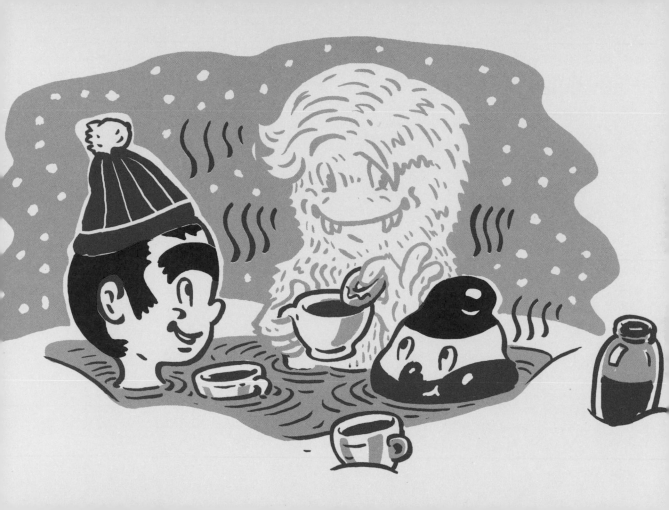

HOT COCOA KEBOB

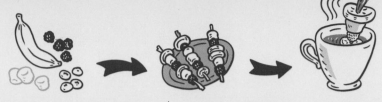

If you are going to go to the trouble of finding natural hot springs to melt your cramps, you may as well have a killer hot cocoa recipe to go along for the ride. And if you are going to go to the trouble of getting a killer hot cocoa recipe, you might as well use mine—Vinnie's Hot Cocoa Kebob.

Kebobs are popularly known as skewers of chopped veggies and meat prepared for summer BBQs. I've borrowed this cool summertime concept to create a hot wintertime treat using cinnamon sticks, marshmallows, bananas, and berries. Simply load the marshmallows and chopped fruit onto the cinnamon-stick kebob and dip into a hot, steaming mug of cocoa. Enjoy as the combined flavors tantalize your taste buds (and as the heat puts the freeze on your cramps!).

YOU WILL NEED:

FOR THE KEBOBS

8–12 large marshmallows

12–16 raspberries

1 banana, cut into 8 chunks

4 slender 6-inch cinnamon sticks (or long coffee stirrers or 5-inch bamboo skewers)

FOR THE COCOA

1/4 cup unsweetened cocoa

1/2 cup sugar

1/3 cup hot water

1/8 teaspoon salt

4 cups low-fat milk

3/4 teaspoon vanilla

* Make the kebobs by spearing the marshmallows, berries, and bananas pieces on the cinnamon sticks in any arrangement you like. Set the kebobs aside.
* To make the cocoa, stir together the cocoa, sugar, water, and salt in a saucepan.
* Over medium heat, stir constantly until the mixture boils. Use a wire whisk if you have one.
* Cook, stirring constantly, for 1 minute.
* Add the milk and stir over medium until hot, but do not let boil.
* Remove from the heat and add the vanilla; blend well.
* Pour into your favorite mugs and add 1 Cocoa Kebob to each drink.
* Serve 'em up!

MAKES 4 SERVINGS

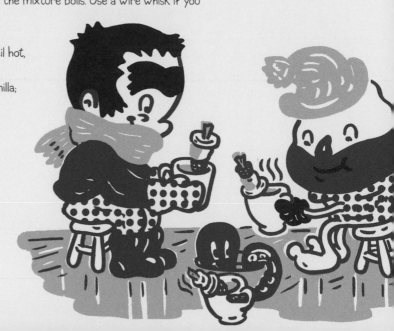

PALM PRESS FOR CRAMP-CURING SUCCESS

There will be times when you won't have easy access to your favorite cramp remedies. Being on a ski lift twenty feet in the air is one of those times. This is when you will want to have committed a few choice remedies to memory—just in case of these precarious occasions. The Palm Press is a simple remedy to remember and E-Z enough to perform on a precarious ski lift, but works great even when you are on the ground.

According to certain scientists and palm readers, our hands actually have points in them that directly relate to other parts of our body. Since this is a cramp-remedy book, you'll be intrigued to know that the bottom part of your palm directly relates to your hip and pelvic region—the home and hangout of those pesky crazy cramps.

HERE'S HOW IT WORKS.
* First, you'll need an assistant. Being on a ski lift is perfect because you are almost always sitting next to someone and you both have time on your hands—and hands are all you need for the Palm Press. (If you are not on a ski lift, the Palm Press is perfect for performing at slumber parties.)
* Take off your ski glove and put your hand out, palm-side up.

* Have your assistant take one of your hands in both of their hands (see diagram A).
* Have them place their thumbs on the lower part of your palm and rub in circles (see diagram B). They can press down as hard as you feel comfortable. Have them rub in circles for a couple minutes.
* Switch hands.
* Before you know it, a tingly sensation will surround your cramps and they will suddenly vanish. Or something like that.

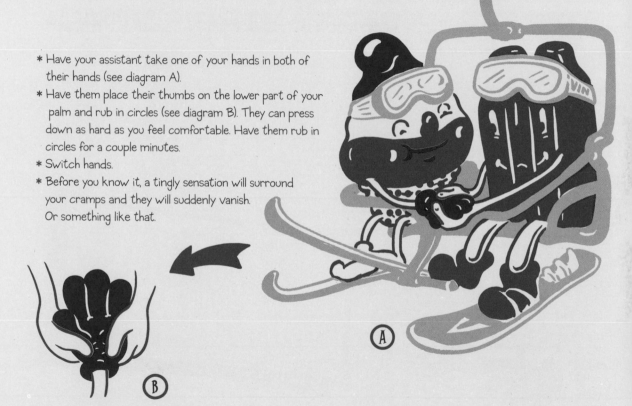

SKYE'S PEANUT BUTTER COOKIE AND PRETZEL SANDWICH

Here's a custom remedy sent in by "Sugar-N-Salt" Skye that combines the benefits of literature, calcium, pretzels, and finely chopped legumes.

PURCHASE THE FOLLOWING:
Peanut butter cookies (preferably soft)
Pretzel sticks (not braids, not rings, not nubs, not bits, not heart shaped—STICKS!)
Skim milk (1 quart will do nicely for a lone cramp sufferer; 1 quart per sufferer is my ratio)
Trashiest magazine possible

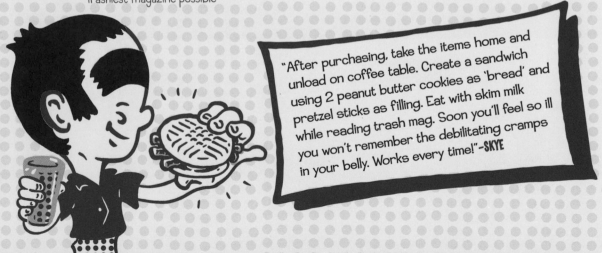

"After purchasing, take the items home and unload on coffee table. Create a sandwich using 2 peanut butter cookies as 'bread' and pretzel sticks as filling. Eat with skim milk while reading trash mag. Soon you'll feel so ill you won't remember the debilitating cramps in your belly. Works every time!" -SKYE

ALL-MIXED-UP TEA PARTY

Other than warming you up after a day of tearing up the slopes, a steaming hot mug of herbal tea can also banish your cramps all the way to the other side of the mountain.

But which tea is truly the best when it comes to relieving even the most crazy cramps? Chamomile? Peppermint? Cramp Bark?!!! (It's real—I didn't make this up! Look for it in health food stores.) Everybody claims their favorite flavor is the cramp-curing champ. This battle for the best brew rages on! Why debate when you can throw an impromptu All-Mixed-Up Tea Party instead? Simply combine everyone's favorite tea into one teapot, steep, and serve.

YOU WILL NEED:

3 cups water
½ teaspoon peppermint tea leaves
½ teaspoon dried chamomile
½ teaspoon ground ginger
½ teaspoon raspberry leaf tea leaves
½ teaspoon cramp bark
Lemon slices
Honey to taste

* Bring the water to a boil.
* Combine all the tea in a tea ball or reusable cotton tea bag.
* Place the tea ball or bag in a teapot and pour in the boiling water. Let steep for 5–10 minutes, depending on how strong you like it.
* Pour into your favorite mugs and add the lemon slices and honey.

MAKES 2 SERVINGS

HOT VINN CUSTOM WATER-BOTTLE COZY

In prehistoric times, cave women used something called a hot-water bottle to relieve their crazy cramps. This thick rubber container with a screw-on top wasn't very sleek, but it worked magic when placed on the tummy of cramping cave teens as they made cave paintings or sat on the couch waiting for video games to be invented. Too bad cramps didn't become extinct along with the dang dinosaurs.

Hot-water bottles survived the Ice Age and are still around because when it comes to melting menstrual cramps, their portable heat is nearly unbeatable. It's time to give this cramp-curing ceratosaurus a second chance and a new look.

This furry Hot Vinn cozy cover for the hot-water bottle will be your hot and comfy companion on the couch as it melts your cramps. Place it on your tummy or put this high-Fahrenheit fur ball behind you to heat up your aching lower back as you play the video games the cave teens coveted.

YOU WILL NEED:

- Two 19-by-9-inch pieces of red furry fabric
- Pencil or pen
- Straight pins
- Scissors
- Needle and black and red thread
- One 6½-by-2-inch piece of black furry fabric or felt
- One 8-inch piece of ¼-inch-wide Velcro
- Hot-water bottle

* Lay 1 piece of the red fabric, furry-side down, on a table, along with this book open to this page.
* With the pencil or pen, draw the outline of Hot Vinn's head on the back of the fabric, comfortably close to the edges (i.e., big enough to hold the hot-water bottle).
* Pin together the 2 pieces of red fabric, furry-sides in.
* Cut along your drawn line so you cut the same shape out of both pieces of fabric (see diagram A).
* Cut a fat eyebrow shape out of the black fabric (see diagram B).
* Remove the pins from the red fabric pieces, and sew the black eyebrow, furry-side up, onto the furry side of one of the red headpieces of fabric (see diagram C), using the black thread.
* Fold over ¼ inch of the neck edge of one edge piece so that the fur is showing. Sew this in place with the red thread. Repeat with the neck edge of the second red piece.
* Using red thread, sew the hooked half of the Velcro along one folded furry edge and the fuzzy half of the Velcro on the other; trim any extra Velcro (see diagram D).
* Finish the job by placing the red fabric pieces on top of each other again, still furry-side in, and stitching with red thread to close the whole shape (except for the Velcro opening at the bottom—Hot Vinn's neck), about ¼ inch from the edge (see diagram E).
* Turn it inside out and voila—it's ready to roll.
* Insert hot-water bottle into your new Hot Vinn Custom Water-Bottle Cozy and get ready for some cozy comfort!

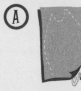

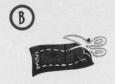

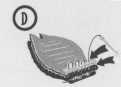

LIVE KITTY HEAT PAD

How cool would it be to have a heating pad that would come when you called its name and readily jump onto your lap to melt your cramps while you read your favorite book by the crackling fire in the ski lodge (or at home with your feet up on the heater)?

This is not a sci-fi fantasy at all, my period-having pal, but a cramp-curing reality that might just be lying around the lodge as we speak! That's right, your pet cat is a super-handy heating pad that will readily remind those crazy cramps to scram. All you gotta do is grab a good book, plant yourself in the most comfy seat in the house, and place kitty on your lap. The ever-so-slight vibrations caused by kitty's purring is an added cramp-relieving bonus.

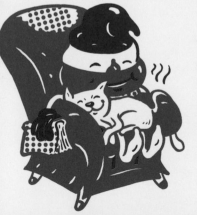

"Dear Vinnie, This always works for me when my cramps are kickin'!! Get some vanilla or chocolate soy milk and put it in a pan. Heat it up, burn it even for that campfire feeling. Get an enormous and lazy cat. Give him or her some of the warm soy milk. Find a chair or couch where you can lean back, place the now real groggy and content cat on your achy ovaries, sip the potion, and watch something on the tube that won't make you laugh too hard. Continually pet the cat to keep it put and purring if your chosen cat is particularly squirrelly. Love ya!"- **NIKKI**

HOT HAND TUMMY RUB

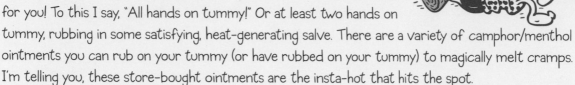

On a chilly day, when you want to cold-clock your cramps, you'll want to reach for the fast heat. Better yet, have the fast heat reach for you! To this I say, "All hands on tummy!" Or at least two hands on tummy, rubbing in some satisfying, heat-generating salve. There are a variety of camphor/menthol ointments you can rub on your tummy (or have rubbed on your tummy) to magically melt cramps. I'm telling you, these store-bought ointments are the insta-hot that hits the spot.

It's like having an out-of-control wildfire swirl around on top of your tummy. It's like having an out-of-control wildfire swirl around on top of your tummy while fire-breathing dragons breathe their fiery breath on your belly. It's like having an out-of-control wildfire swirl around on top of your tummy while fire-breathing dragons breathe their fiery breath on your belly as a single hot, freshly baked doughnut falls off the doughnut truck right onto the crampiest spot on your tummy.

NOW, THAT SPELLS R-E-L-I-E-F!

* Get a tube of heat-generating salve (available at most pharmacies and grocery stores).
* Apply salve to the crampy area of your tummy yourself, or enlist a pal to help.

NOTE: Be sure to keep the salve out of your eyes and do not put on food. Heat salves do not work to heat up leftover pizza.

CHART-N-CHILL

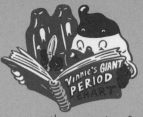

It's one thing to come up with a variety of remedies to combat your cramps and PMS, but it's even better to be able to predict 'em before they happen. To do this you can either make a Psychic Snowball to forecast your next menstrual cycle or you can keep track of your period on a regular calendar.

Psychic Snowballs require a fresh snowfall, packing a snowball the size of a softball, and sticking this snowball in the freezer for twenty-four hours. Then there's something about casting a spell on the snowball with uncooked asparagus and sprinkling olive oil on it. Personally, I think you're better off with the period chart. Charting your monthly cycle is E-Z.

HERE'S HOW TO DO IT:

* Get a calendar (or use my **GIANT ROLLER COASTER PERIOD CHART & JOURNAL STICKER BOOK**)
* Mark down on the calendar various aspects of your monthly cycle as they happen so you can begin to track the pattern from month to month:

    1. every day you experience PMS

    2. every day of your period

    3. crazy-cramp days

    4. heavy-flow days

    5. tender-boob days

* Keep track of your remedy schedule as well:
  1. calcium days (milk shakes, spinach, or baked tofu cookies 4 days before your next period)
  2. exercise days
  3. massage appointments
* Leave your period chart out for everyone to see it. Your brother can watch for the days he needs to be EXTRA nice to you, maybe make you brownies (try Aunt Fran's Red-Hot Brownies, page 52, or a Cramp-Curin' Kiwi Shake, page 17). Turns out everybody benefits when they know about your monthly cycle—especially you.

Each month you'll be able to look back and see the similarities and a pattern will soon emerge. A few months down the road your chart will give you an idea of how many days you deal with PMS, how many days your actual period lasts, and which days you usually are rocked by the crazy cramps.

The more you know about what to expect and when to expect it, the better prepared you'll be to take care of yourself.

KNOW YOUR FLOW!

SLED O' ICE CREAM EXERCISE

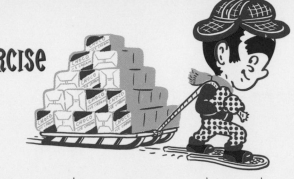

EXERCISE.

ICE CREAM.

EXERCISE.

ICE CREAM.

Exercise and ice cream are so rarely seen in the same sentence much less in the same cramp remedy—until now! Exercise from a full day of sledding will reward you with a healthy appetite, a cheery disposition, and a supersound sleep. Ice cream soothes the soul, doubles as a cure for the bubonic plague, wards off stray asteroids in the solar system, and makes your tummy real happy. Since both make you feel really good it only makes sense to combine them and double the fun, right? Right.

* The first thing you are going to need is a really big sled. Dig one out of the garage and grab some skate wax while you're at it.
* Turn the sled over and, with a soft cloth, rub the skate wax onto the blades of the sled.
* Next go back into the garage and get your snowshoes. If you have some wax left over, maybe wax up the snowshoes.

* Hop on the sled and take off downhill toward town. The wax on the blades should make the sled glide through the snow like hot corn through butter or a Hot Vinn Deluxe (page 92) through cramps.
* Steer toward your local grocery store.
* Park your sled out front.
* Go into the store and buy all of their ice cream. ALL of it.
* Have your pal who bags groceries give you a hand stacking the ice cream on your sled. You might want to bring some rope or a bungee cord to strap all that ice cream onto the sled.
* Put on your snowshoes, get a good grip on the tow rope, and start your trek home. This is where the real exercise starts (sledding downhill on the way to the store barely counts as exercise, duh!).

Pulling a half a ton of ice cream up a steep hill in deep snow is REALLY good exercise. The rewards here are very obvious:

* Regular exercise is a great way to keep your cramps at bay.
* Having hundreds of containers of ice cream on hand, in case of emergency or in case of a case of crazy cramps, is very important.
* You can build an ice-cream container igloo in your yard. Have a sleepover with your pals.

FRO-ZEN REPOSE-ZEN

Whether you have been outside all day building an igloo or whether you are experiencing polar-bear-size cramps, it's important to take a moment to defrost. Defrosting is the time a frozen pizza sits on the kitchen counter outside the freezer and before you chuck it into the heated oven. You should take a similar break between excessive activity in the frozen tundra and before you get heated up balancing your checkbook.

The Fro-Zen Repose-Zen is the perfect yoga pose for defrosting, as well as for relieving lower-back pain from lifting too many ice blocks or from crazy menstrual cramps. I recommend you take off the snowsuit and the snow boots for this.

* Find a large bolster (a couch cushion or two pillows from the bed).
* Snag the all-purpose towel from the Burrito Lumbar-Support Device (page 14) and fold it in quarters.

* Lay the bolster on the floor and put the folded towel on one end as extra support for your head.
* Lie back on the bolster so one end rests in the curve of your lower back and the back of your head is on the folded towel.
* Bring the bottoms of your feet together and let your knees flop comfortably to the sides. You can put rolled-up towels under each knee for extra support and comfort.
* Let your arms flop along your sides, palms facing up.
* Relax and rest this way for 5–10 minutes.

Be good to your body and your body will be good to you back.

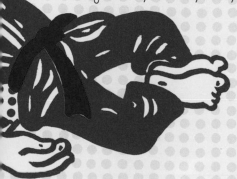

HOT VINN DELUXE

Wouldn't it be great to have a reliable and ever-ready Period Pal who would massage your crampy tummy and sit on the couch next to you as you watch some dorky movie? Well, if Dr. Frankenstein could fashion a monster out of spare parts found in the basement, the least you can do is create a friend and masseuse from a pair of old socks and some rice. Right? Right.

Introducing the Hot Vinn Deluxe. This sensational sock solution is a ready cure for stubborn cramps—simply sew him up and chuck him into the microwave. And when he's not cramp crunching, prop him up on the couch and you have a ready companion to suffer through any movie you toss in the player.

YOU WILL NEED:

1 pair of red socks (preferably 100% cotton)
Scissors
Needle and thread
One 2½-by-1-inch piece of black felt

2 buttons
5 cups dry rice or flaxseed
   (don't use instant rice)
A handful of cotton balls

* Cut off the toe of one sock (see diagram A).
* Cut the top 4 inches of the sock in half vertically (see diagram B).
* Create the Vinnie flame hair by cutting the toe end and sew Hot Vinn's legs closed (see diagram C).

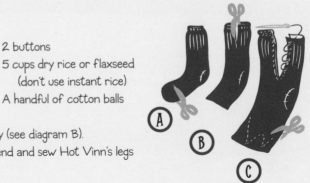

* Cut out an eyebrow shape from the black felt.
* Sew the eyebrow and button eyes below the flaming hair to make the face (see diagram D).
* Stitch a smile below the eyes with contrasting thread (see diagram D again).
* Stitch closed about three-quarters of the flame-hair seam, leaving an opening three fingers wide (see diagram E).
* Pour in as much rice or flaxseed as needed to make a hearty Hot Vinn (see diagram E again).
* Finish sewing Hot Vinn closed.
* Cut the top off of the second sock about 3½ inches down from the leg hole of the sock and cut that tube in half to make the arms (see diagram F).
* Sew the arms along the long sides, stuff with cotton balls, and stitch the ends closed.
* Sew the arms onto the body (see diagram G).
* Toss the Hot Vinn Deluxe into the microwave for about 2 minutes. Remove from the microwave and place on your tummy (be sure Hot Vinn isn't too hot. Let him cool down a tad or put a towel or shirt between your tummy and Hot Vinn if necessary).
* Relax on the couch as Hot Vinn melts your cramps!

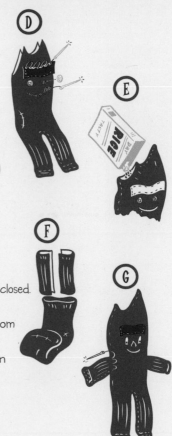

93

Remedy Reminder Charm Bracelet

You know you've been there. You've eaten half of a chocolate cake while crying at a '70s ice-skating movie on TV. Your pal comes into the kitchen and simply stares at your chocolate-covered face. He knows what's up even if you have forgotten: PMS.

So the cake was for his hockey team's bake sale—you were under the influence of PMS. Even with the best intentions and a methodically filled-out period chart (page 86), you might still experience irrational behavior such as unexplainable outbursts of tears or the sudden and unprovoked attack on a defenseless yet delicious chocolate cake.

To remind you, as you cry and shovel cake into your mouth, that you are merely in the midst of your monthly cycle, make a Remedy Reminder Charm Bracelet. Wiping tears on your sleeve, you will catch sight of the jangly bracelet and be reminded of the reality of the situation and that, in fact, you don't particularly like '70s skating movies, or at least not this one.

Once you are reminded, you can take the appropriate steps to take care of yourself (i.e., relaxing, taking a warm bath, exercising, getting a massage, or eating the rest of the cake now that it can no longer be used for the bake sale).

YOU WILL NEED:

Lettered or numbered beads (available at most fabric stores
   or department stores)

String or elasticized string

Other colored or decorative beads to fill out the bracelet

* With your lettered beads, spell out a word or message that will instantly remind you what it is you need to relax or be comfortable during your monthly cycle (and to remind your pals what they can do to transform you back into a happier state). This is a great excuse to channel your inner poet and be abstract and creative. Ideas:

   * Spell out your favorite remedy: Hot Vinn Deluxe, bubbles, H_2O, kiwi shake, cake, etc.
   * Spell out the name of your favorite Period Pal (i.e., Vinnie) so you remember to call him for support.
   * The phone number of your gynecologist.

* String your lettered or numbered beads, adding decorative beads to fill the bracelet out, and tie it off.

* Slip the bracelet over your wrist when your period chart says IT'S PMS TIME.

* Bake another cake for your pal to bring to his bake sale.

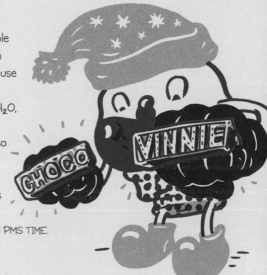

BEANBAG BOOTY BEND

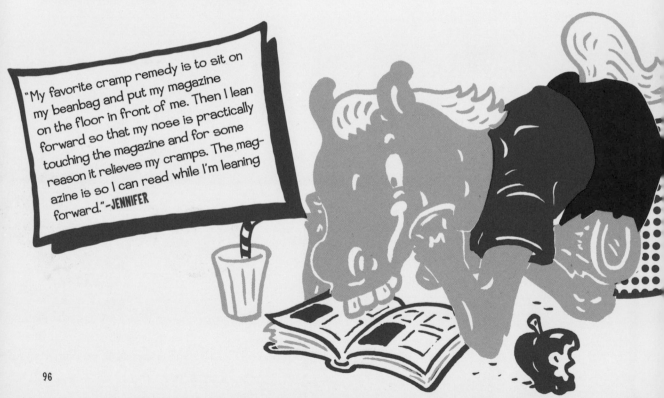

"My favorite cramp remedy is to sit on my beanbag and put my magazine on the floor in front of me. Then I lean forward so that my nose is practically touching the magazine and for some reason it relieves my cramps. The magazine is so I can read while I'm leaning forward." -JENNIFER

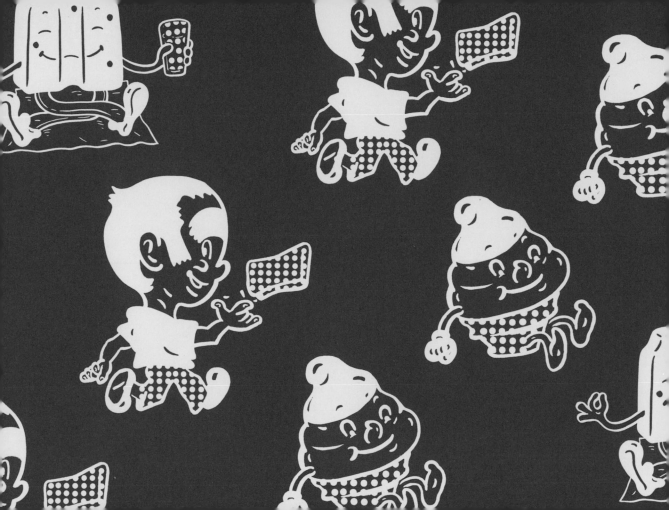

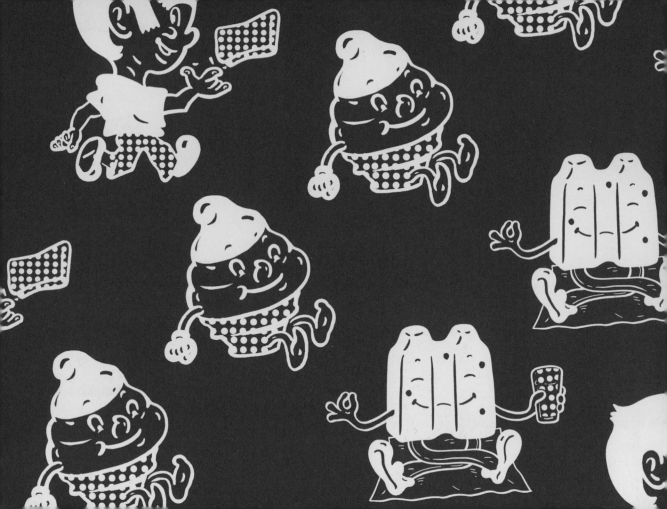